LOW-CARB DOG FOOD AND TREATS COOKBOOK

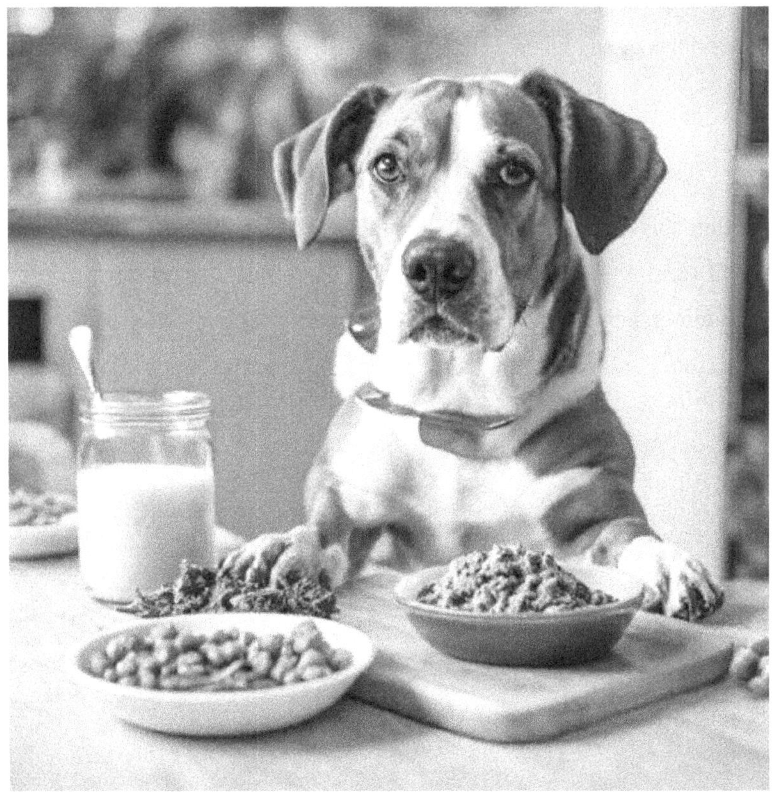

Dr. Wesley Glasgow

TABLE OF CONTENTS

INTRODUCTION

My journey into the world of canine nutrition began with a simple act of love. As a lifelong dog lover, my childhood was enriched by the presence of my first canine companion, Dan. From the moment Dan entered my life, he became more than just a pet; he was my loyal friend, confidant, and source of boundless joy.

Dan was more than just a pet; he was family. And like any devoted pet owner, I wanted to give him the best of everything. From premium kibble to gourmet treats, I showered Dan with indulgences, believing that I was showing him love through food. Little did I know, my well-intentioned gestures were setting him on a path to poor health.

Years passed, and despite my love and care, Dan's health began to deteriorate. He became lethargic, overweight, and developed a host of health issues. It wasn't until a routine visit to the veterinarian revealed the devastating truth – Dan had been diagnosed with diabetes. My heart sank as I realized that my beloved companion was suffering because of my ignorance about proper canine nutrition.

With the guidance of our trusted veterinarian, Dan's diet underwent a radical transformation. Gone were the days of indulgence and excess; instead, Dan's meals were carefully crafted to meet his nutritional needs and manage his condition. Witnessing the remarkable turnaround in Dan's health opened my eyes to the transformative power of good nutrition.

From that moment on, I dedicated myself to learning everything I could about canine nutrition. I pursued a career in veterinary medicine, driven by a passion to help other dogs live their healthiest, happiest lives. Over the years, I honed my skills in the kitchen, experimenting with recipes and ingredients to create meals that were not only delicious but also nourishing for our furry friends.

Today, as a seasoned veterinarian and accomplished cook, I am proud to present this low-carb dog food and treats cookbook. Each recipe has been meticulously tested and approved by me, ensuring that every bite is packed with flavor and goodness. But don't just take my word for it – I've shared these recipes with family, friends, and patients alike, all of whom have experienced the transformative benefits of healthy eating for their dogs.

In this cookbook, you'll find a collection of mouthwatering recipes designed to tantalize your dog's taste buds while supporting their overall health and well-being. From savory main courses to delectable treats, each recipe is crafted with love and care, using wholesome ingredients that are low in carbs and high in nutrition.

But this cookbook is more than just a collection of recipes – it's a guide to better health for your beloved pet. Throughout these pages, you'll discover the benefits of healthy eating for dogs, as well as the dangers and consequences of unhealthy eating habits. You'll learn how proper nutrition can improve your dog's energy levels, maintain a healthy weight, and even prevent common health issues like diabetes and obesity.

By incorporating the recipes in this cookbook into your dog's diet, you'll not only be treating them to delicious meals but also giving them the gift of a longer, happier life. So, join me on this journey to unleash your dog's health and vitality – one nutritious meal at a time.

Together, let's nourish our dogs from the inside out and give them the love and care they deserve.

Contact the Author

Thank you for reading my book! I would love to hear from you, whether you have feedback, questions, or just want to share your thoughts. Your feedback means a lot to me and helps me improve as a writer.

Please don't hesitate to reach out to me through

glasgowesley@gmail.com

I look forward to connecting with my readers and appreciate your support in this literary journey. Your thoughts and comments are valuable to me.

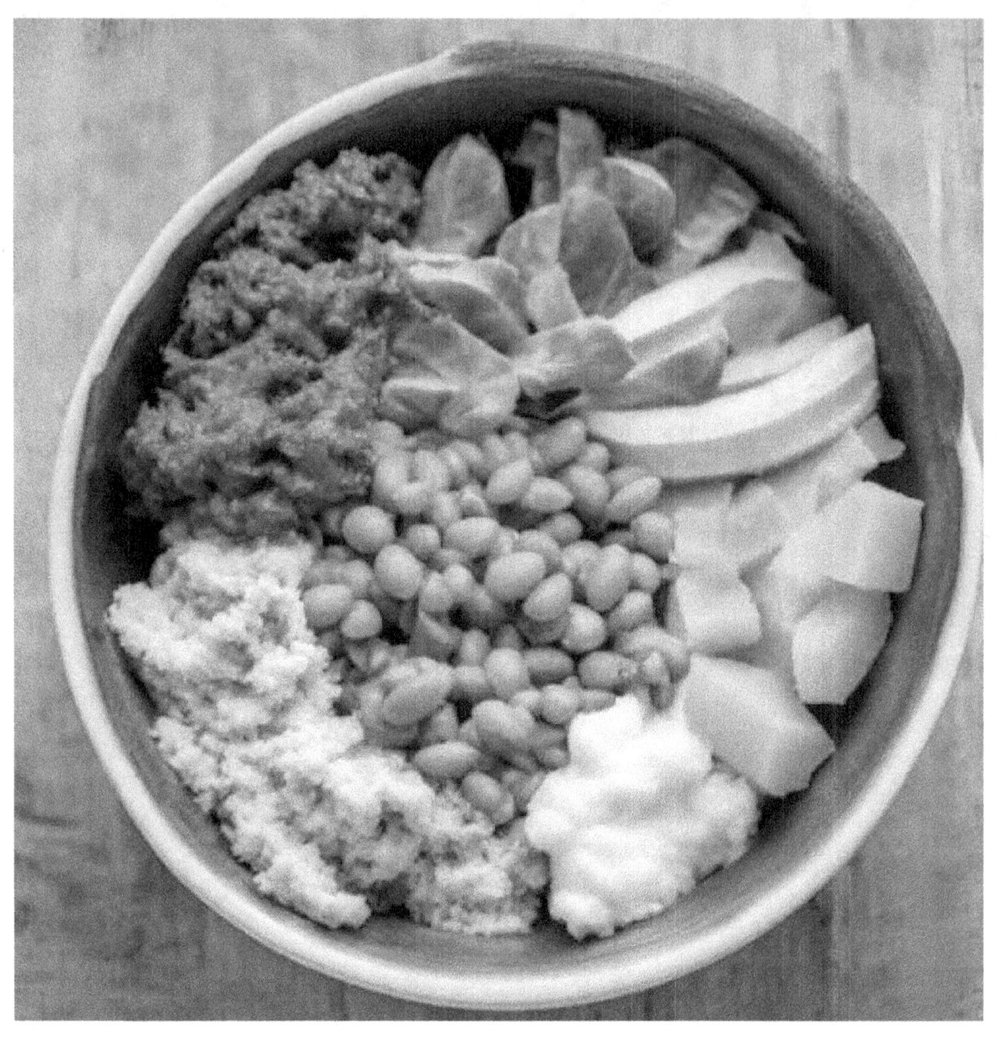

CHAPTER 1
Understanding Canine Nutrition

When it comes to ensuring the health and vitality of our canine companions, understanding their nutritional needs is paramount. Just like humans, dogs require a balanced diet comprised of essential nutrients to support their overall well-being. From carbohydrates to proteins, fats, and micronutrients, each component plays a crucial role in maintaining optimal health for our furry friends.

Essential Nutrients for Dogs

Essential nutrients are those that dogs must obtain from their diet as their bodies cannot produce them in sufficient quantities. These include proteins, fats, carbohydrates, vitamins, and minerals. Providing a balanced diet that incorporates these nutrients in appropriate proportions is fundamental for supporting your dog's growth, energy levels, immune function, and overall health.

Carbohydrates in Dog Food: What You Need to Know

Carbohydrates are a primary source of energy for dogs. While they are not considered essential in the same way as proteins and fats, they still play a valuable role in providing fuel for physical activity and supporting digestive health. Common sources of carbohydrates in dog food include grains like rice, oats, and barley, as well as vegetables such as sweet potatoes and peas. It's essential to select carbohydrates that are easily digestible and provide necessary fiber for digestive regularity.

Protein Requirements for Dogs

Proteins are crucial for building and repairing tissues, supporting muscle development, and maintaining a healthy immune system. High-quality sources of protein in dog food include meat, poultry, fish, eggs, and legumes. It's important to ensure that your dog's diet contains sufficient protein content, especially for active dogs, puppies, and lactating females, as their requirements may be higher.

Fats and Oils: The Good, the Bad, and the Essential

Fats and oils are essential for dogs as they provide concentrated energy, support nutrient absorption, and contribute to healthy skin and coat. However, not all fats are created equal. While some fats are beneficial, others, such as trans fats, can be harmful to canine health. Incorporating sources of omega-3 and omega-6 fatty acids, such as fish oil and flaxseed oil, can promote cardiovascular health and reduce inflammation in dogs.

Micronutrients: Vitamins and Minerals for Canine Health

Micronutrients, including vitamins and minerals, play vital roles in various physiological processes within a dog's body. These include bone development, immune function, and metabolic reactions. Common vitamins and minerals essential for dogs include vitamin A, vitamin D, vitamin E, calcium, phosphorus, and zinc. While commercial dog foods are formulated to meet these requirements, supplementation may be necessary in certain cases, such as specific health conditions or dietary restrictions.

CHAPTER 2

Getting Started with Low Carb Cooking for Dogs

Embarking on the journey of low carb cooking for your canine companion is a rewarding Endeavor that can enhance their health and vitality. Whether you're looking to manage your dog's weight, address health issues, or simply provide a nutritionally balanced diet, understanding the basics of low carb cooking is essential. Here's a guide to help you get started:

Tools and Equipment You'll Need:

1. **Quality Food Processor or Blender**: A reliable food processor or blender is indispensable for chopping, blending, and pureeing ingredients to the desired consistency for your dog's meals.

2. **Kitchen Scale**: Accurate measurement of ingredients is crucial for maintaining proper portion sizes and nutritional balance. A kitchen scale helps ensure consistency and precision in your recipes.

3. **Stainless Steel Cookware**: Invest in high-quality stainless-steel pots and pans for cooking your dog's meals. Stainless steel is durable, easy to clean, and doesn't leach harmful chemicals into food.

4. **Sharp Chef's Knife**: A sharp chef's knife makes chopping vegetables, meat, and other ingredients a breeze. Choose a knife that feels comfortable and secure in your hand for safe and efficient meal preparation.

5. **Food Storage Containers**: Opt for airtight food storage containers to safely store homemade dog food in the refrigerator or freezer. Glass or BPA-free

plastic containers are ideal for maintaining freshness and preventing contamination.

Ingredients: Choosing the Best for Your Dog

When selecting ingredients for your dog's low carb meals, focus on high-quality, nutrient-rich foods that meet their dietary needs. Here are some key ingredients to include:

1. **Lean Protein Sources**: Choose lean cuts of meat such as chicken, turkey, beef, or fish as the primary protein source in your dog's meals. Protein is essential for muscle growth, repair, and overall health.

2. **Low Carb Vegetables**: Incorporate non-starchy vegetables like spinach, broccoli, cauliflower, and green beans into your dog's meals to add fiber, vitamins, and minerals without excess carbohydrates.

3. **Healthy Fats**: Include sources of healthy fats such as olive oil, coconut oil, or fatty fish like salmon or sardines to provide essential omega-3 fatty acids for skin, coat, and joint health.

4. **Low Glycaemic Fruits**: While fruits should be limited due to their sugar content, small amounts of berries such as blueberries or raspberries can be added for flavour and antioxidants.

5. **Supplements**: Consider adding dog-safe supplements like calcium, vitamin D, or omega-3 fatty acids to ensure your dog receives all the essential nutrients they need for optimal health.

Safety Guidelines for Preparing Homemade Dog Food

Follow these safety guidelines to ensure the health and safety of your dog when preparing homemade low carb meals:

1. **Consult with Your Veterinarian**: Before making any dietary changes or introducing new foods to your dog's diet, consult with your veterinarian to ensure it's appropriate for their age, breed, and health status.

2. **Maintain Proper Hygiene**: Wash your hands, utensils, and food preparation surfaces thoroughly before and after handling raw ingredients to prevent contamination and foodborne illness.

3. **Avoid Harmful Ingredients**: Steer clear of ingredients that are toxic to dogs, such as onions, garlic, grapes, raisins, chocolate, and xylitol. These substances can be harmful or even fatal to dogs if ingested.

4. **Monitor Portion Sizes**: Pay attention to portion sizes and calorie intake to prevent overfeeding and weight gain. Use your dog's weight, activity level, and nutritional needs as a guide when determining serving sizes.

5. **Transition Gradually**: When transitioning your dog to a new diet, gradually introduce new foods over the course of several days to prevent digestive upset or food aversions.

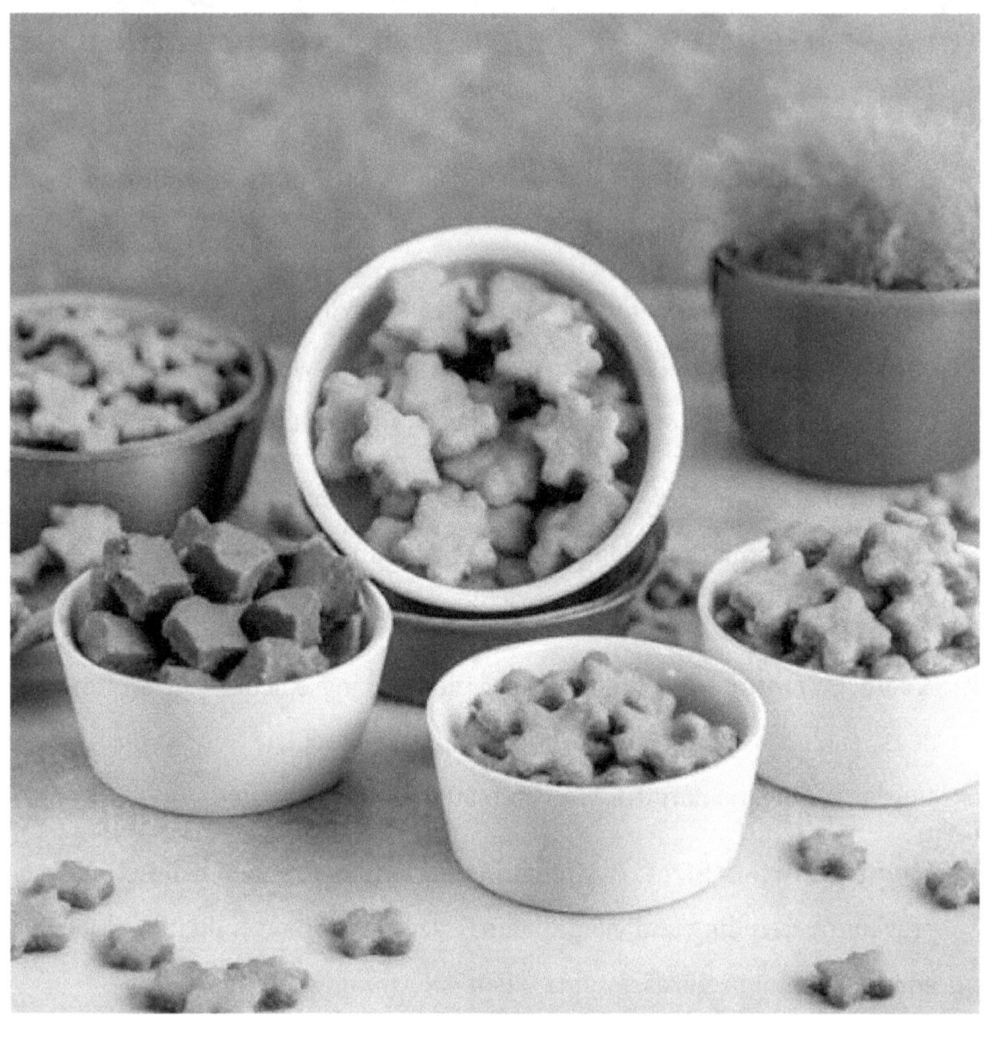

CHAPTER 3

Homemade Low-Carb Treats

Baked Chicken and Sweet Potato Bites

Cooking Time: 25 minutes

Servings: 12 treats

Ingredients:

- 1 boneless, skinless chicken breast
- 1 small sweet potato, peeled and diced
- 1 egg

Instructions:

1. Preheat your oven to 350°F (175°C).

2. Boil or steam the sweet potato until tender, then mash it thoroughly.

3. Cook the chicken breast until fully cooked, then finely chop or shred it.

4. In a bowl, mix together the mashed sweet potato, chopped chicken, and egg until well combined.

5. Scoop small portions of the mixture onto a baking sheet lined with parchment paper, shaping them into bite-sized treats.

6. Bake in the preheated oven for 15-20 minutes or until the treats are firm and lightly browned.

7. Allow them to cool completely before serving.

Nutritional Information: Per serving - Calories: 45, Protein: 5g, Fat: 1g, Carbohydrates: 3g, Fiber: 1g

Peanut Butter and Pumpkin Balls

Cooking Time: 20 minutes

Servings: 10 treats

Ingredients:

- 1/2 cup canned pumpkin puree
- 1/4 cup natural peanut butter (no added sugar or salt)
- 1/4 cup coconut flour
- 1 egg

Instructions:

1. Preheat your oven to 350°F (175°C) and line a baking sheet with parchment paper.

2. In a mixing bowl, combine the pumpkin puree, peanut butter, coconut flour, and egg until a thick dough forms.

3. Roll the dough into small balls and place them on the prepared baking sheet.

4. Flatten each ball slightly with a fork.

5. Bake in the preheated oven for 12-15 minutes or until the treats are firm and lightly golden.

6. Allow them to cool completely before serving.

Nutritional Information: Per serving - Calories: 50, Protein: 2g, Fat: 3g, Carbohydrates: 3g, Fiber: 1g

Tuna and Cheese Crunchies

Cooking Time: 30 minutes

Servings: 15 treats

Ingredients:

- 1 can tuna in water, drained

- 1/2 cup shredded cheddar cheese

- 1/2 cup almond flour

- 1 egg

Instructions:

1. Preheat your oven to 350°F (175°C) and line a baking sheet with parchment paper.

2. In a mixing bowl, combine the drained tuna, shredded cheese, almond flour, and egg until well mixed.

3. Form the mixture into small balls or shapes and place them on the prepared baking sheet.

4. Flatten each ball slightly with your fingers or a fork.

5. Bake in the preheated oven for 20-25 minutes or until the treats are golden brown and crunchy.

6. Allow them to cool completely before serving.

Nutritional Information: Per serving - Calories: 55, Protein: 4g, Fat: 3g, Carbohydrates: 1g, Fiber: 0.5g

Zucchini and Chicken Jerky

Cooking Time: 3 hours

Servings: 20 treats

Ingredients:

- 1 large zucchini

- 1 boneless, skinless chicken breast

Instructions:

1. Preheat your oven to the lowest setting (around 170°F or 75°C).

2. Slice the zucchini and chicken breast into thin strips.

3. Place the slices on a baking sheet lined with parchment paper, making sure they don't overlap.

4. Bake in the preheated oven for 2-3 hours, flipping halfway through, until the slices are dried and crunchy.

5. Let them cool completely before serving. Store in an airtight container.

Nutritional Information: Per serving - Calories: 25, Protein: 3g, Fat: 1g, Carbohydrates: 1g, Fiber: 0.5g

Blueberry and Coconut Bites

Cooking Time: 25 minutes

Servings: 12 treats

Ingredients:

- 1/2 cup coconut flour

- 1/4 cup unsweetened applesauce

- 1/4 cup fresh blueberries, mashed

- 1 egg

Instructions:

1. Preheat your oven to 350°F (175°C) and line a baking sheet with parchment paper.

2. In a mixing bowl, combine the coconut flour, applesauce, mashed blueberries, and egg until a dough forms.

3. Roll the dough into small balls and place them on the prepared baking sheet.

4. Flatten each ball slightly with your fingers or a fork.

5. Bake in the preheated oven for 15-20 minutes or until the treats are firm and lightly golden.

6. Allow them to cool completely before serving.

Nutritional Information: Per serving - Calories: 40, Protein: 2g, Fat: 2g, Carbohydrates: 3g, Fiber: 1.5g

Turkey and Spinach Patties

Cooking Time: 20 minutes

Servings: 8 treats

Ingredients:

- 1/2 lb ground turkey

- 1 cup fresh spinach, chopped

- 1/4 cup almond flour

- 1 egg

Instructions:

1. Preheat your oven to 350°F (175°C) and line a baking sheet with parchment paper.

2. In a mixing bowl, combine the ground turkey, chopped spinach, almond flour, and egg until well mixed.

3. Form the mixture into small patties and place them on the prepared baking sheet.

4. Bake in the preheated oven for 15-20 minutes or until the patties are cooked through.

5. Allow them to cool completely before serving.

Nutritional Information: Per serving - Calories: 65, Protein: 6g, Fat: 4g, Carbohydrates: 1g, Fiber: 0.5g

Carrot and Chicken Biscuits

Cooking Time: 30 minutes

Servings: 12 treats

Ingredients:

- 1/2 cup cooked chicken, shredded

- 1/2 cup grated carrot

- 1/4 cup coconut flour

- 1 egg

Instructions:

1. Preheat your oven to 350°F (175°C) and line a baking sheet with parchment paper.

2. In a mixing bowl, combine the shredded chicken, grated carrot, coconut flour, and egg until a dough forms.

3. Roll out the dough on a floured surface to about 1/4-inch thickness.

4. Use cookie cutters to cut out shapes or simply slice into small squares.

5. Place the biscuits on the prepared baking sheet.

6. Bake in the preheated oven for 20-25 minutes or until the treats are firm and lightly browned.

7. Allow them to cool completely before serving.

Nutritional Information: Per serving - Calories: 40, Protein: 3g, Fat: 2g, Carbohydrates: 2g, Fiber: 1g

Salmon and Pea Cookies

Cooking Time: 25 minutes

Servings: 10 treats

Ingredients:

- 1/2 cup canned salmon, drained and mashed

- 1/4 cup cooked peas, mashed

- 1/4 cup almond flour

- 1 egg

Instructions:

1. Preheat your oven to 350°F (175°C) and line a baking sheet with parchment paper.

2. In a mixing bowl, combine the mashed salmon, mashed peas, almond flour, and egg until well mixed.

3. Roll out the dough on a floured surface to about 1/4-inch thickness.

4. Use cookie cutters to cut out shapes or simply slice into small squares.

5. Place the cookies on the prepared baking sheet.

6. Bake in the preheated oven for 15-20 minutes or until the treats are firm and lightly browned.

7. Allow them to cool completely before serving.

Nutritional Information: Per serving - Calories: 50, Protein: 4g, Fat: 3g, Carbohydrates: 1.5g, Fiber: 0.5g

Beef and Broccoli Bites

Cooking Time: 30 minutes

Servings: 12 treats

Ingredients:

- 1/2 lb lean ground beef

- 1/2 cup finely chopped broccoli florets

- 1/4 cup coconut flour

- 1 egg

Instructions:

1. Preheat your oven to 350°F (175°C) and line a baking sheet with parchment paper.

2. In a mixing bowl, combine the ground beef, chopped broccoli, coconut flour, and egg until well mixed.

3. Roll the mixture into small balls and place them on the prepared baking sheet.

4. Flatten each ball slightly with your fingers or a fork.

5. Bake in the preheated oven for 20-25 minutes or until the treats are cooked through.

6. Allow them to cool completely before serving.

Nutritional Information: Per serving - Calories: 55, Protein: 5g, Fat: 3g, Carbohydrates: 2g, Fiber: 1g

Apple and Turkey Roll-Ups

Cooking Time: 20 minutes

Servings: 8 treats

Ingredients:

- 1/2 lb sliced turkey breast
- 1 apple, thinly sliced
- 1/4 cup unsweetened applesauce

Instructions:

1. Preheat your oven to 350°F (175°C) and line a baking sheet with parchment paper.

2. Lay out the turkey slices on a clean surface.

3. Spread a thin layer of unsweetened applesauce onto each turkey slice.

4. Place an apple slice on one end of each turkey slice and roll it up tightly.

5. Secure the roll-ups with toothpicks if necessary.

6. Place the roll-ups on the prepared baking sheet.

7. Bake in the preheated oven for 15-20 minutes or until the turkey is cooked through.

8. Allow them to cool slightly before serving.

Nutritional Information: Per serving - Calories: 45, Protein: 5g, Fat: 1g, Carbohydrates: 3g, Fiber: 0.5g

Cheese and Bacon Biscuits

Cooking Time: 25 minutes

Servings: 12 treats

Ingredients:

- 1 cup almond flour

- 1/2 cup shredded cheddar cheese

- 2 slices cooked bacon, crumbled

- 1 egg

Instructions:

1. Preheat your oven to 350°F (175°C) and line a baking sheet with parchment paper.

2. In a mixing bowl, combine the almond flour, shredded cheese, crumbled bacon, and egg until a dough forms.

3. Roll out the dough on a floured surface to about 1/4-inch thickness.

4. Use cookie cutters to cut out shapes or simply slice into small squares.

5. Place the biscuits on the prepared baking sheet.

6. Bake in the preheated oven for 20-25 minutes or until the treats are firm and lightly browned.

7. Allow them to cool completely before serving.

Nutritional Information: Per serving - Calories: 70, Protein: 4g, Fat: 5g, Carbohydrates: 2g, Fiber: 1g

Pumpkin and Turkey Meatballs

Cooking Time: 30 minutes

Servings: 12 treats

Ingredients:

- 1/2 cup canned pumpkin puree

- 1/2 lb ground turkey

- 1/4 cup coconut flour

- 1 egg

Instructions:

1. Preheat your oven to 350°F (175°C) and line a baking sheet with parchment paper.

2. In a mixing bowl, combine the pumpkin puree, ground turkey, coconut flour, and egg until well mixed.

3. Roll the mixture into small meatballs and place them on the prepared baking sheet.

4. Bake in the preheated oven for 25-30 minutes or until the meatballs are cooked through.

5. Allow them to cool slightly before serving.

Nutritional Information: Per serving - Calories: 55, Protein: 4g, Fat: 3g, Carbohydrates: 2g, Fiber: 1g

Spinach and Cheese Squares

Cooking Time: 20 minutes

Servings: 12 treats

Ingredients:

- 1 cup cooked spinach, chopped

- 1/2 cup shredded mozzarella cheese

- 1/4 cup coconut flour

- 1 egg

Instructions:

1. Preheat your oven to 350°F (175°C) and line a baking sheet with parchment paper.

2. In a mixing bowl, combine the cooked spinach, shredded mozzarella cheese, coconut flour, and egg until well mixed.

3. Spread the mixture evenly onto the prepared baking sheet.

4. Bake in the preheated oven for 15-20 minutes or until the mixture is set and lightly browned.

5. Allow it to cool slightly, then cut into squares before serving.

Nutritional Information: Per serving - Calories: 45, Protein: 3g, Fat: 3g, Carbohydrates: 1g, Fiber: 0.5g

Beef and Liver Jerky

Cooking Time: 4 hours

Servings: 15 treats

Ingredients:

- 1/2 lb beef liver

- 1/2 lb lean beef steak

Instructions:

1. Preheat your oven to the lowest setting (around 170°F or 75°C).

2. Slice the beef liver and beef steak into thin strips.

3. Place the strips on a baking sheet lined with parchment paper, making sure they don't overlap.

4. Bake in the preheated oven for 3-4 hours, flipping halfway through, until the strips are dried and chewy.

5. Let them cool completely before serving. Store in an airtight container.

Nutritional Information: Per serving - Calories: 50, Protein: 6g, Fat: 2g, Carbohydrates: 0g, Fiber: 0g

Carrot and Oatmeal Cookies

Cooking Time: 25 minutes

Servings: 12 treats

Ingredients:

- 1/2 cup grated carrot

- 1/2 cup rolled oats

- 1/4 cup unsweetened applesauce

- 1 egg

Instructions:

1. Preheat your oven to 350°F (175°C) and line a baking sheet with parchment paper.

2. In a mixing bowl, combine the grated carrot, rolled oats, unsweetened applesauce, and egg until well mixed.

3. Drop spoonful's of the dough onto the prepared baking sheet, spacing them apart.

4. Flatten each cookie slightly with your fingers.

5. Bake in the preheated oven for 15-20 minutes or until the cookies are firm and lightly browned.

6. Allow them to cool completely before serving.

Nutritional Information: Per serving - Calories: 35, Protein: 2g, Fat: 1g, Carbohydrates: 4g, Fiber: 1g

Turkey and Cranberry Balls

Cooking Time: 20 minutes

Servings: 10 treats

Ingredients:

- 1/2 lb ground turkey

- 1/4 cup dried cranberries, chopped

- 1/4 cup almond flour

- 1 egg

Instructions:

1. Preheat your oven to 350°F (175°C) and line a baking sheet with parchment paper.

2. In a mixing bowl, combine the ground turkey, chopped dried cranberries, almond flour, and egg until well mixed.

3. Roll the mixture into small balls and place them on the prepared baking sheet.

4. Bake in the preheated oven for 15-20 minutes or until the treats are cooked through.

5. Allow them to cool slightly before serving.

Nutritional Information: Per serving - Calories: 60, Protein: 5g, Fat: 3g, Carbohydrates: 2g, Fiber: 0.5g

Green Bean and Chicken Chips

Cooking Time: 3 hours

Servings: 20 treats

Ingredients:

- 1/2 lb boneless, skinless chicken breast

- 1 cup fresh green beans, trimmed

Instructions:

1. Preheat your oven to the lowest setting (around 170°F or 75°C).

2. Slice the chicken breast and green beans into thin strips.

3. Place the strips on a baking sheet lined with parchment paper, making sure they don't overlap.

4. Bake in the preheated oven for 2-3 hours, flipping halfway through, until the strips are dried and crunchy.

5. Let them cool completely before serving. Store in an airtight container.

Nutritional Information: Per serving - Calories: 25, Protein: 3g, Fat: 0.5g, Carbohydrates: 1g, Fiber: 0.5g

Salmon and Sweet Potato Slices

Cooking Time: 30 minutes

Servings: 15 treats

Ingredients:

- 1/2 lb salmon fillet, skin removed

- 1 small sweet potato, thinly sliced

Instructions:

1. Preheat your oven to 350°F (175°C) and line a baking sheet with parchment paper.

2. Slice the salmon fillet into thin strips.

3. Place the salmon strips and sweet potato slices on the prepared baking sheet, ensuring they don't overlap.

4. Bake in the preheated oven for 20-25 minutes or until the treats are cooked through and the sweet potatoes are crispy.

5. Let them cool completely before serving.

Nutritional Information: Per serving - Calories: 40, Protein: 4g, Fat: 2g, Carbohydrates: 1.5g, Fiber: 0.5g

Coconut and Carrot Balls

Cooking Time: 20 minutes

Servings: 10 treats

Ingredients:

- 1/2 cup shredded carrot

- 1/4 cup unsweetened shredded coconut

- 1/4 cup coconut flour

- 1 egg

Instructions:

1. Preheat your oven to 350°F (175°C) and line a baking sheet with parchment paper.

2. In a mixing bowl, combine the shredded carrot, shredded coconut, coconut flour, and egg until a dough forms.

3. Roll the dough into small balls and place them on the prepared baking sheet.

4. Flatten each ball slightly with your fingers.

5. Bake in the preheated oven for 15-20 minutes or until the treats are firm and lightly browned.

6. Allow them to cool completely before serving.

Nutritional Information: Per serving - Calories: 45, Protein: 2g, Fat: 3g, Carbohydrates: 2g, Fiber: 1g

Chicken and Green Pea Patties

Cooking Time: 25 minutes

Servings: 8 treats

Ingredients:

- 1/2 lb ground chicken
- 1/2 cup cooked green peas, mashed
- 1/4 cup almond flour
- 1 egg

Instructions:

1. Preheat your oven to 350°F (175°C) and line a baking sheet with parchment paper.

2. In a mixing bowl, combine the ground chicken, mashed green peas, almond flour, and egg until well mixed.

3. Form the mixture into small patties and place them on the prepared baking sheet.

4. Bake in the preheated oven for 20-25 minutes or until the patties are cooked through.

5. Allow them to cool slightly before serving.

Nutritional Information: Per serving - Calories: 70, Protein: 6g, Fat: 4g, Carbohydrates: 2g, Fiber: 1g

Chicken and Carrot Sticks

Cooking Time: 25 minutes

Servings: 10 treats

Ingredients:

- 1 boneless, skinless chicken breast

- 1 large carrot, peeled and cut into sticks

Instructions:

1. Preheat your oven to 350°F (175°C) and line a baking sheet with parchment paper.

2. Cut the chicken breast into thin strips.

3. Wrap each carrot stick with a strip of chicken.

4. Place the wrapped carrot sticks on the prepared baking sheet.

5. Bake in the preheated oven for 20-25 minutes or until the chicken is cooked through.

6. Allow them to cool slightly before serving.

Nutritional Information: Per serving - Calories: 40, Protein: 6g, Fat: 1g, Carbohydrates: 2g, Fiber: 1g

Beef and Pumpkin Jerky

Cooking Time: 4 hours

Servings: 15 treats

Ingredients:

- 1/2 lb lean beef steak

- 1/2 cup canned pumpkin puree

Instructions:

1. Preheat your oven to the lowest setting (around 170°F or 75°C).

2. Slice the beef steak into thin strips.

3. Spread a thin layer of pumpkin puree onto each strip of beef.

4. Place the strips on a baking sheet lined with parchment paper, making sure they don't overlap.

5. Bake in the preheated oven for 3-4 hours, flipping halfway through, until the strips are dried and chewy.

6. Let them cool completely before serving. Store in an airtight container.

Nutritional Information: Per serving - Calories: 55, Protein: 7g, Fat: 2g, Carbohydrates: 2g, Fiber: 0.5g

Salmon and Cucumber Slices

Cooking Time: 15 minutes

Servings: 10 treats

Ingredients:

- 1/2 lb salmon fillet, skin removed

- 1 small cucumber, thinly sliced

Instructions:

1. Preheat your oven to 350°F (175°C) and line a baking sheet with parchment paper.

2. Cut the salmon fillet into thin slices.

3. Place a slice of cucumber on each salmon slice and roll it up.

4. Place the roll-ups on the prepared baking sheet.

5. Bake in the preheated oven for 12-15 minutes or until the salmon is cooked through.

6. Allow them to cool slightly before serving.

Nutritional Information: Per serving - Calories: 45, Protein: 6g, Fat: 2g, Carbohydrates: 1g, Fiber: 0.5g

Turkey and Zucchini Chips

Cooking Time: 3 hours

Servings: 20 treats

Ingredients:

- 1/2 lb ground turkey

- 1 large zucchini, thinly sliced

Instructions:

1. Preheat your oven to the lowest setting (around 170°F or 75°C).

2. Season the ground turkey as desired.

3. Place a small amount of ground turkey on each zucchini slice.

4. Place the slices on a baking sheet lined with parchment paper.

5. Bake in the preheated oven for 2-3 hours, flipping halfway through, until the turkey is cooked through and the zucchini is dried.

6. Let them cool completely before serving. Store in an airtight container.

Nutritional Information: Per serving - Calories: 35, Protein: 4g, Fat: 1g, Carbohydrates: 1g, Fiber: 0.5g

Beef and Green Bean Rolls

Cooking Time: 25 minutes

Servings: 10 treats

Ingredients:

- 1/2 lb lean beef steak

- 1 cup fresh green beans, trimmed

Instructions:

1. Preheat your oven to 350°F (175°C) and line a baking sheet with parchment paper.

2. Cut the beef steak into thin strips.

3. Place a green bean on each beef strip and roll it up.

4. Place the rolls on the prepared baking sheet.

5. Bake in the preheated oven for 20-25 minutes or until the beef is cooked through.

6. Allow them to cool slightly before serving.

Nutritional Information: Per serving - Calories: 60, Protein: 8g, Fat: 2g, Carbohydrates: 2g, Fiber: 1g

Chicken and Broccoli Bites

Cooking Time: 30 minutes

Servings: 12 treats

Ingredients:

- 1 boneless, skinless chicken breast

- 1 cup cooked broccoli, finely chopped

Instructions:

1. Preheat your oven to 350°F (175°C) and line a baking sheet with parchment paper.

2. Cook the chicken breast until fully cooked, then finely chop or shred it.

3. In a mixing bowl, combine the cooked chicken and chopped broccoli until well mixed.

4. Form the mixture into small balls and place them on the prepared baking sheet.

5. Flatten each ball slightly with your fingers or a fork.

6. Bake in the preheated oven for 20-25 minutes or until the treats are cooked through.

7. Allow them to cool completely before serving.

Nutritional Information: Per serving - Calories: 40, Protein: 6g, Fat: 1g, Carbohydrates: 2g, Fiber: 1g

Turkey and Cauliflower Nuggets

Cooking Time: 25 minutes

Servings: 12 treats

Ingredients:

- 1/2 lb ground turkey
- 1 cup cooked cauliflower, mashed
- 1/4 cup almond flour
- 1 egg

Instructions:

1. Preheat your oven to 350°F (175°C) and line a baking sheet with parchment paper.

2. In a mixing bowl, combine the ground turkey, mashed cauliflower, almond flour, and egg until well mixed.

3. Form the mixture into small nuggets and place them on the prepared baking sheet.

4. Bake in the preheated oven for 20-25 minutes or until the treats are cooked through.

5. Allow them to cool slightly before serving.

Nutritional Information: Per serving - Calories: 50, Protein: 5g, Fat: 2g, Carbohydrates: 2g, Fiber: 1g

Salmon and Carrot Rounds

Cooking Time: 20 minutes

Servings: 10 treats

Ingredients:

- 1/2 lb salmon fillet, skin removed

- 1 large carrot, thinly sliced

Instructions:

1. Preheat your oven to 350°F (175°C) and line a baking sheet with parchment paper.

2. Cut the salmon fillet into thin slices.

3. Place a slice of carrot on each salmon slice.

4. Place the rounds on the prepared baking sheet.

5. Bake in the preheated oven for 15-20 minutes or until the salmon is cooked through.

6. Allow them to cool slightly before serving.

Nutritional Information: Per serving - Calories: 50, Protein: 6g, Fat: 2g, Carbohydrates: 1g, Fiber: 0.5g

Chicken and Green Pea Balls

Cooking Time: 25 minutes

Servings: 12 treats

Ingredients:

- 1 boneless, skinless chicken breast

- 1/2 cup cooked green peas, mashed

Instructions:

1. Preheat your oven to 350°F (175°C) and line a baking sheet with parchment paper.

2. Cook the chicken breast until fully cooked, then finely chop or shred it.

3. In a mixing bowl, combine the cooked chicken and mashed green peas until well mixed.

4. Form the mixture into small balls and place them on the prepared baking sheet.

5. Flatten each ball slightly with your fingers or a fork.

6. Bake in the preheated oven for 20-25 minutes or until the treats are cooked through.

7. Allow them to cool completely before serving.

Nutritional Information: Per serving - Calories: 40, Protein: 6g, Fat: 1g, Carbohydrates: 2g, Fiber: 1g

Beef and Asparagus Rolls

Cooking Time: 25 minutes

Servings: 10 treats

Ingredients:

- 1/2 lb lean beef steak
- 10 asparagus spears, trimmed

Instructions:

1. Preheat your oven to 350°F (175°C) and line a baking sheet with parchment paper.

2. Cut the beef steak into thin strips.

3. Place an asparagus spear on each beef strip and roll it up.

4. Place the rolls on the prepared baking sheet.

5. Bake in the preheated oven for 20-25 minutes or until the beef is cooked through.

6. Allow them to cool slightly before serving.

Nutritional Information: Per serving - Calories: 60, Protein: 8g, Fat: 2g, Carbohydrates: 1g, Fiber: 0.5g

CHAPTER 4
Low-Carb Breakfast option

Egg and Spinach Scramble

Cooking Time: 10 minutes

Servings: 1 serving

Ingredients:

- 2 eggs

- 1/4 cup fresh spinach, chopped

Instructions:

1. Heat a non-stick skillet over medium heat.

2. Crack the eggs into a bowl and whisk until well beaten.

3. Pour the eggs into the skillet and let them cook for a minute.

4. Add the chopped spinach to the eggs and gently stir.

5. Continue cooking until the eggs are fully cooked and the spinach is wilted.

6. Remove from heat and let it cool slightly before serving.

Nutritional Information: Calories: 140, Protein: 12g, Fat: 9g, Carbohydrates: 2g, Fiber: 1g

Chicken and Cheese Omelette

Cooking Time: 15 minutes

Servings: 1 serving

Ingredients:

- 2 eggs

- 1/4 cup cooked chicken, shredded

- 1/4 cup shredded cheddar cheese

Instructions:

1. Beat the eggs in a bowl until well mixed.

2. Heat a non-stick skillet over medium heat and pour in the beaten eggs.

3. Let the eggs cook for a minute, then sprinkle the shredded chicken and cheese evenly over one half of the omelette.

4. Gently fold the other half of the omelette over the filling.

5. Cook for another 2-3 minutes until the cheese is melted and the omelette is cooked through.

6. Allow it to cool slightly before serving.

Nutritional Information: Calories: 270, Protein: 25g, Fat: 17g, Carbohydrates: 1g, Fiber: 0.5g

Turkey and Vegetable Frittata

Cooking Time: 20 minutes

Servings: 2 servings

Ingredients:

- 4 eggs

- 1/2 cup cooked turkey, diced

- 1/4 cup diced bell peppers

- 1/4 cup diced zucchini

- 1/4 cup diced tomatoes

Instructions:

1. Preheat your oven to 350°F (175°C).

2. In a bowl, beat the eggs until well mixed.

3. Stir in the diced turkey, bell peppers, zucchini, and tomatoes.

4. Pour the mixture into a greased oven-safe skillet.

5. Bake in the preheated oven for 15-20 minutes or until the frittata is set and golden brown.

6. Allow it to cool slightly before serving.

Nutritional Information: Calories: 220, Protein: 20g, Fat: 12g, Carbohydrates: 4g, Fiber: 1.5g

Salmon and Sweet Potato Hash

Cooking Time: 25 minutes

Servings: 2 servings

Ingredients:

- 1/2 lb cooked salmon, flaked

- 1 small sweet potato, peeled and diced

- 1/4 cup diced red onion

- 1/4 cup diced bell peppers

Instructions:

1. Heat a skillet over medium heat and add a small amount of oil.

2. Add the diced sweet potato to the skillet and cook until slightly softened, about 5 minutes.

3. Add the diced red onion and bell peppers to the skillet and cook for another 3-4 minutes.

4. Stir in the flaked salmon and cook for an additional 2-3 minutes until heated through.

5. Remove from heat and let it cool slightly before serving.

Nutritional Information: Calories: 250, Protein: 22g, Fat: 10g, Carbohydrates: 16g, Fiber: 2.5g

Turkey and Spinach Breakfast Muffins

Cooking Time: 30 minutes

Servings: 6 muffins

Ingredients:

- 4 eggs

- 1/2 cup cooked turkey, diced

- 1/4 cup chopped spinach

- 1/4 cup shredded cheddar cheese

Instructions:

1. Preheat your oven to 350°F (175°C) and grease a muffin tin.

2. In a bowl, beat the eggs until well mixed.

3. Stir in the diced turkey, chopped spinach, and shredded cheddar cheese.

4. Pour the mixture evenly into the muffin tin compartments.

5. Bake in the preheated oven for 20-25 minutes or until the muffins are set and lightly golden.

6. Allow them to cool slightly before serving.

Nutritional Information: Calories: 150, Protein: 12g, Fat: 10g, Carbohydrates: 1g, Fiber: 0.5g

Beef and Broccoli Breakfast Bowl

Cooking Time: 20 minutes

Servings: 2 servings

Ingredients:

- 1/2 lb cooked lean beef, diced

- 1 cup cooked broccoli florets

- 2 eggs, cooked to preference

Instructions:

1. Divide the cooked beef and broccoli evenly into two bowls.

2. Top each bowl with a cooked egg.

3. Serve immediately, allowing the egg yolk to act as a sauce when broken.

Nutritional Information: Calories: 320, Protein: 30g, Fat: 15g, Carbohydrates: 6g, Fiber: 3g

Turkey and Pumpkin Breakfast Casserole

Cooking Time: 40 minutes

Servings: 4 servings

Ingredients:

- 1/2 lb cooked turkey, diced

- 1 cup canned pumpkin puree

- 4 eggs

- 1/4 cup shredded mozzarella cheese

Instructions:

1. Preheat your oven to 350°F (175°C) and grease a baking dish.

2. In a bowl, mix together the cooked turkey and pumpkin puree until well combined.

3. Spread the mixture evenly in the prepared baking dish.

4. In another bowl, beat the eggs until well mixed.

5. Pour the beaten eggs over the turkey and pumpkin mixture.

6. Sprinkle the shredded mozzarella cheese on top.

7. Bake in the preheated oven for 25-30 minutes or until the casserole is set and the cheese is melted and bubbly.

8. Allow it to cool slightly before serving.

Nutritional Information: Calories: 280, Protein: 25g, Fat: 14g, Carbohydrates: 8g, Fiber: 2g

Chicken and Vegetable Breakfast Skillet

Cooking Time: 25 minutes

Servings: 2 servings

Ingredients:

- 1/2 lb cooked chicken breast, diced

- 1 cup diced sweet potatoes

- 1/2 cup diced bell peppers

- 1/4 cup diced red onion

Instructions:

1. Heat a skillet over medium heat and add a small amount of oil.

2. Add the diced sweet potatoes to the skillet and cook until slightly softened, about 5 minutes.

3. Add the diced bell peppers and red onion to the skillet and cook for another 3-4 minutes.

4. Stir in the diced chicken breast and cook for an additional 2-3 minutes until heated through.

5. Remove from heat and let it cool slightly before serving.

Nutritional Information: Calories: 320, Protein: 30g, Fat: 5g, Carbohydrates: 25g, Fiber: 4g

Beef and Spinach Breakfast Wraps

Cooking Time: 15 minutes

Servings: 2 servings

Ingredients:

- 4 large lettuce leaves

- 1/2 lb cooked lean beef, thinly sliced

- 1/4 cup chopped spinach

- 1/4 cup diced tomatoes

Instructions:

1. Lay out the lettuce leaves on a clean surface.

2. Divide the cooked beef, chopped spinach, and diced tomatoes evenly among the lettuce leaves.

3. Roll up each lettuce leaf to form a wrap.

4. Serve immediately.

Nutritional Information: Calories: 240, Protein: 25g, Fat: 10g, Carbohydrates: 5g, Fiber: 2g

Salmon and Asparagus Breakfast Bake

Cooking Time: 30 minutes

Servings: 4 servings

Ingredients:

- 1/2 lb cooked salmon, flaked

- 1 cup cooked asparagus, chopped

- 4 eggs

- 1/4 cup shredded cheddar cheese

Instructions:

1. Preheat your oven to 350°F (175°C) and grease a baking dish.

2. Spread the cooked salmon and chopped asparagus evenly in the prepared baking dish.

3. In a bowl, beat the eggs until well mixed.

4. Pour the beaten eggs over the salmon and asparagus mixture.

5. Sprinkle the shredded cheddar cheese on top.

6. Bake in the preheated oven for 20-25 minutes or until the bake is set and the cheese is melted and bubbly.

7. Allow it to cool slightly before serving.

Nutritional Information: Calories: 280, Protein: 25g, Fat: 15g, Carbohydrates: 4g, Fiber: 1.5g

CHAPTER 5

Low-Carb Main Courses

Chicken and Vegetable Stir-Fry

Cooking Time: 20 minutes

Servings: 2 servings

Ingredients:

- 1/2 lb boneless, skinless chicken breast, thinly sliced
- 1 cup mixed vegetables (such as broccoli, carrots, and bell peppers), chopped
- 1 tablespoon olive oil

Instructions:

1. Heat the olive oil in a skillet over medium-high heat.

2. Add the sliced chicken breast to the skillet and cook until browned and cooked through, about 5-7 minutes.

3. Remove the chicken from the skillet and set aside.

4. In the same skillet, add the chopped vegetables and stir-fry until tender-crisp, about 3-5 minutes.

5. Add the cooked chicken back to the skillet and toss to combine with the vegetables.

6. Remove from heat and let it cool slightly before serving.

Nutritional Information: Calories: 250, Protein: 25g, Fat: 10g, Carbohydrates: 8g, Fiber: 3g

Turkey and Cauliflower Rice Bowl

Cooking Time: 25 minutes

Servings: 2 servings

Ingredients:

- 1/2 lb ground turkey
- 2 cups cauliflower florets
- 1/4 cup diced tomatoes
- 1 tablespoon coconut oil

Instructions:

1. Pulse the cauliflower florets in a food processor until they resemble rice grains.

2. Heat the coconut oil in a skillet over medium heat.

3. Add the ground turkey to the skillet and cook until browned and cooked through, about 5-7 minutes.

4. Remove the cooked turkey from the skillet and set aside.

5. In the same skillet, add the cauliflower rice and diced tomatoes.

6. Stir-fry until the cauliflower is tender, about 5-7 minutes.

7. Add the cooked turkey back to the skillet and mix well.

8. Remove from heat and let it cool slightly before serving.

Nutritional Information: Calories: 280, Protein: 30g, Fat: 12g, Carbohydrates: 10g, Fiber: 4g

Salmon and Green Bean Bake

Cooking Time: 30 minutes

Servings: 2 servings

Ingredients:

- 1/2 lb salmon fillet, cut into cubes

- 1 cup fresh green beans, trimmed

- 1 tablespoon olive oil

Instructions:

1. Preheat your oven to 350°F (175°C) and grease a baking dish.

2. Place the salmon cubes and green beans in the baking dish.

3. Drizzle with olive oil and toss to coat evenly.

4. Bake in the preheated oven for 20-25 minutes or until the salmon is cooked through and the green beans are tender.

5. Let it cool slightly before serving.

Nutritional Information: Calories: 300, Protein: 25g, Fat: 15g, Carbohydrates: 8g, Fiber: 4g

Beef and Spinach Meatballs

Cooking Time: 25 minutes

Servings: 2 servings

Ingredients:

- 1/2 lb ground beef

- 1 cup chopped spinach

- 1 egg

Instructions:

1. Preheat your oven to 375°F (190°C) and line a baking sheet with parchment paper.

2. In a bowl, mix together the ground beef, chopped spinach, and egg until well combined.

3. Form the mixture into small meatballs and place them on the prepared baking sheet.

4. Bake in the preheated oven for 20-25 minutes or until cooked through.

5. Let them cool slightly before serving.

Nutritional Information: Calories: 280, Protein: 30g, Fat: 15g, Carbohydrates: 2g, Fiber: 1g

Turkey and Pumpkin Stew

Cooking Time: 30 minutes

Servings: 2 servings

Ingredients:

- 1/2 lb cooked turkey, shredded

- 1 cup canned pumpkin puree

- 1/2 cup low-sodium chicken broth

Instructions:

1. In a pot, combine the shredded turkey, pumpkin puree, and chicken broth.

2. Stir well to combine.

3. Bring the mixture to a simmer over medium heat.

4. Reduce the heat to low and let the stew cook for 20-25 minutes, stirring occasionally.

5. Let it cool slightly before serving.

Nutritional Information: Calories: 250, Protein: 25g, Fat: 10g, Carbohydrates: 10g, Fiber: 3g

Chicken and Sweet Potato Casserole

Cooking Time: 40 minutes

Servings: 2 servings

Ingredients:

- 1/2 lb boneless, skinless chicken breast, diced

- 1 large sweet potato, peeled and diced

- 1/4 cup low-sodium chicken broth

Instructions:

1. Preheat your oven to 375°F (190°C) and grease a baking dish.

2. Place the diced chicken breast and sweet potato in the baking dish.

3. Pour the chicken broth over the chicken and sweet potato.

4. Cover the baking dish with foil and bake in the preheated oven for 30-35 minutes or until the chicken is cooked through and the sweet potato is tender.

5. Let it cool slightly before serving.

Nutritional Information: Calories: 280, Protein: 30g, Fat: 5g, Carbohydrates: 20g, Fiber: 3g

Beef and Broccoli Stir-Fry

Cooking Time: 20 minutes

Servings: 2 servings

Ingredients:

- 1/2 lb lean beef steak, thinly sliced

- 2 cups broccoli florets

- 2 tablespoons soy sauce (low-sodium)

Instructions:

1. Heat a skillet over medium-high heat.

2. Add the sliced beef steak to the skillet and cook until browned, about 3-5 minutes.

3. Remove the beef from the skillet and set aside.

4. In the same skillet, add the broccoli florets and soy sauce.

5. Stir-fry until the broccoli is tender-crisp, about 3-5 minutes.

6. Add the cooked beef back to the skillet and toss to combine.

7. Remove from heat and let it cool slightly before serving.

Nutritional Information: Calories: 280, Protein: 30g, Fat: 10g, Carbohydrates: 10g, Fiber: 4g

Salmon and Zucchini Skewers

Cooking Time: 15 minutes

Servings: 2 servings

Ingredients:

- 1/2 lb salmon fillet, cut into chunks

- 1 zucchini, sliced into rounds

- Wooden skewers, soaked in water

Instructions:

1. Preheat your grill to medium heat.

2. Thread the salmon chunks and zucchini rounds onto the skewers.

3. Grill the skewers for 6-8 minutes, turning occasionally, until the salmon is cooked through and the zucchini is tender.

4. Let them cool slightly before serving.

Nutritional Information: Calories: 300, Protein: 25g, Fat: 15g, Carbohydrates: 6g, Fiber: 2g

Turkey and Carrot Meatloaf

Cooking Time: 45 minutes

Servings: 4 servings

Ingredients:

- 1/2 lb ground turkey

- 1 carrot, grated

- 1 egg

Instructions:

1. Preheat your oven to 375°F (190°C) and grease a loaf pan.

2. In a bowl, mix together the ground turkey, grated carrot, and egg until well combined.

3. Transfer the mixture to the prepared loaf pan and press it down evenly.

4. Bake in the preheated oven for 35-40 minutes or until cooked through.

5. Let it cool slightly before serving.

Nutritional Information: Calories: 200, Protein: 20g, Fat: 10g, Carbohydrates: 5g, Fiber: 1g

Beef and Green Bean Casserole

Cooking Time: 35 minutes

Servings: 2 servings

Ingredients:

- 1/2 lb lean beef, diced

- 1 cup green beans, trimmed and chopped

- 1/2 cup low-sodium beef broth

Instructions:

1. Preheat your oven to 375°F (190°C) and grease a baking dish.

2. Place the diced beef and green beans in the baking dish.

3. Pour the beef broth over the beef and green beans.

4. Cover the baking dish with foil and bake in the preheated oven for 25-30 minutes or until the beef is cooked through and the green beans are tender.

5. Let it cool slightly before serving.

Nutritional Information: Calories: 250, Protein: 30g, Fat: 10g, Carbohydrates: 8g, Fiber: 3g

CHAPTER 6

Low-Carb Soups and Stew

Turkey and Vegetable Soup

Cooking Time: 30 minutes

Servings: 4 servings

Ingredients:

- 1/2 lb ground turkey

- 2 cups mixed vegetables (such as carrots, green beans, and peas), diced

- 4 cups low-sodium chicken broth

Instructions:

1. In a pot, brown the ground turkey over medium heat until cooked through.

2. Add the diced vegetables and chicken broth to the pot.

3. Bring the mixture to a boil, then reduce the heat to low and simmer for 20 minutes.

4. Let it cool slightly before serving.

Nutritional Information: Calories: 200, Protein: 20g, Fat: 8g, Carbohydrates: 10g, Fiber: 3g

Beef and Spinach Stew

Cooking Time: 40 minutes

Servings: 4 servings

Ingredients:

- 1/2 lb lean beef stew meat, cubed

- 2 cups fresh spinach leaves

- 1 cup diced tomatoes

- 4 cups low-sodium beef broth

Instructions:

1. In a pot, brown the beef stew meat over medium heat until browned on all sides.

2. Add the diced tomatoes and beef broth to the pot.

3. Bring the mixture to a boil, then reduce the heat to low and simmer for 30 minutes.

4. Stir in the fresh spinach leaves and simmer for an additional 5 minutes.

5. Let it cool slightly before serving.

Nutritional Information: Calories: 220, Protein: 25g, Fat: 10g, Carbohydrates: 8g, Fiber: 2g

Chicken and Pumpkin Soup

Cooking Time: 25 minutes

Servings: 4 servings

Ingredients:

- 1/2 lb boneless, skinless chicken breast, diced

- 1 cup canned pumpkin puree

- 4 cups low-sodium chicken broth

Instructions:

1. In a pot, cook the diced chicken breast over medium heat until cooked through.

2. Add the canned pumpkin puree and chicken broth to the pot.

3. Bring the mixture to a boil, then reduce the heat to low and simmer for 15 minutes.

4. Let it cool slightly before serving.

Nutritional Information: Calories: 180, Protein: 20g, Fat: 5g, Carbohydrates: 10g, Fiber: 3g

Salmon and Sweet Potato Chowder

Cooking Time: 35 minutes

Servings: 4 servings

Ingredients:

- 1/2 lb cooked salmon, flaked

- 2 cups sweet potatoes, peeled and diced

- 4 cups low-sodium vegetable broth

Instructions:

1. In a pot, combine the diced sweet potatoes and vegetable broth.

2. Bring the mixture to a boil, then reduce the heat to low and simmer for 20 minutes or until the sweet potatoes are tender.

3. Add the cooked salmon to the pot and simmer for an additional 5 minutes.

4. Let it cool slightly before serving.

Nutritional Information: Calories: 250, Protein: 25g, Fat: 10g, Carbohydrates: 15g, Fiber: 3g

Turkey and Lentil Stew

Cooking Time: 45 minutes

Servings: 4 servings

Ingredients:

- 1/2 lb ground turkey

- 1 cup lentils, rinsed

- 2 cups mixed vegetables (such as carrots, celery, and peas), diced

- 4 cups low-sodium chicken broth

Instructions:

1. In a pot, brown the ground turkey over medium heat until cooked through.

2. Add the rinsed lentils, diced vegetables, and chicken broth to the pot.

3. Bring the mixture to a boil, then reduce the heat to low and simmer for 30 minutes or until the lentils are tender.

4. Let it cool slightly before serving.

Nutritional Information: Calories: 230, Protein: 20g, Fat: 8g, Carbohydrates: 15g, Fiber: 5g

Beef and Butternut Squash Soup

Cooking Time: 40 minutes

Servings: 4 servings

Ingredients:

- 1/2 lb lean beef stew meat, cubed

- 2 cups butternut squash, peeled and diced

- 4 cups low-sodium beef broth

Instructions:

1. In a pot, brown the beef stew meat over medium heat until browned on all sides.

2. Add the diced butternut squash and beef broth to the pot.

3. Bring the mixture to a boil, then reduce the heat to low and simmer for 30 minutes or until the beef is tender and the squash is soft.

4. Let it cool slightly before serving.

Nutritional Information: Calories: 220, Protein: 25g, Fat: 10g, Carbohydrates: 12g, Fiber: 3g

Chicken and Broccoli Chowder

Cooking Time: 30 minutes

Servings: 4 servings

Ingredients:

- 1/2 lb boneless, skinless chicken breast, diced

- 2 cups broccoli florets

- 4 cups low-sodium chicken broth

Instructions:

1. In a pot, cook the diced chicken breast over medium heat until cooked through.

2. Add the broccoli florets and chicken broth to the pot.

3. Bring the mixture to a boil, then reduce the heat to low and simmer for 15 minutes or until the broccoli is tender.

4. Let it cool slightly before serving.

Nutritional Information: Calories: 180, Protein: 20g, Fat: 5g, Carbohydrates: 10g, Fiber: 3g

Turkey and Vegetable Stew

Cooking Time: 35 minutes

Servings: 4 servings

Ingredients:

- 1/2 lb ground turkey

- 2 cups mixed vegetables (such as carrots, green beans, and zucchini), diced

- 4 cups low-sodium vegetable broth

Instructions:

1. In a pot, brown the ground turkey over medium heat until cooked through.

2. Add the diced vegetables and vegetable broth to the pot.

3. Bring the mixture to a boil, then reduce the heat to low and simmer for 25 minutes.

4. Let it cool slightly before serving.

Nutritional Information: Calories: 200, Protein: 20g, Fat: 8g, Carbohydrates: 12g, Fiber: 4g

Salmon and Cauliflower Soup

Cooking Time: 30 minutes

Servings: 4 servings

Ingredients:

- 1/2 lb cooked salmon, flaked

- 2 cups cauliflower florets

- 4 cups low-sodium vegetable broth

Instructions:

1. In a pot, combine the cauliflower florets and vegetable broth.

2. Bring the mixture to a boil, then reduce the heat to low and simmer for 15 minutes or until the cauliflower is tender.

3. Add the cooked salmon to the pot and simmer for an additional 5 minutes.

4. Let it cool slightly before serving.

Nutritional Information: Calories: 220, Protein: 25g, Fat: 10g, Carbohydrates: 10g, Fiber: 3g

Beef and Cabbage Stew

Cooking Time: 40 minutes

Servings: 4 servings

Ingredients:

- 1/2 lb lean beef stew meat, cubed

- 2 cups cabbage, shredded

- 4 cups low-sodium beef broth

Instructions:

1. In a pot, brown the beef stew meat over medium heat until browned on all sides.

2. Add the shredded cabbage and beef broth to the pot.

3. Bring the mixture to a boil, then reduce the heat to low and simmer for 30 minutes or until the beef is tender and the cabbage is soft.

4. Let it cool slightly before serving.

Nutritional Information: Calories: 220, Protein: 25g, Fat: 10g, Carbohydrates: 10g, Fiber: 3g

<u>OTHER BOOKS BY THE AUTHOR</u>

<u>INSTANT POT DOG FOOD COOKBOOK</u>

<u>DOG FOOD COOKBOOK FOR PICKY EATERS</u>

<u>AIR FRYER DOG FOOD COOKBOOK</u>

<u>SLOW COOKER DOG FOOD COOKBOOK</u>

<u>DOG FOOD COOKBOOK FOR SENSITIVE STOMACH</u>

SCAN THE QR CODE TO SEE MORE BOOKS BY AUTHOR

CONCLUSION

As we come to the end of this culinary journey through the world of low-carb dog food and treats, I hope you feel inspired and empowered to take action for your beloved furry companion. Throughout this cookbook, we've explored a variety of delicious recipes designed to nourish your dog's body and soul, while also promoting their overall health and well-being.

From hearty main courses to irresistible treats, each recipe has been carefully crafted with love and expertise to ensure that every bite is not only delicious but also packed with essential nutrients. By incorporating these recipes into your dog's diet, you'll be providing them with the nourishment they need to thrive – from the inside out.

But our journey doesn't end here. As pet owners, we have a responsibility to continually educate ourselves about proper canine nutrition and to advocate for the health and happiness of our furry friends. I encourage you to share your experiences with these recipes, both the successes and the challenges, as well as any feedback or suggestions you may have.

Your feedback is invaluable in helping us improve and refine our recipes, ensuring that we continue to provide the best possible nutrition for our dogs. So please, don't hesitate to reach out and share your thoughts with us. Together, we can make a difference in the lives of our canine companions and ensure that they live long, healthy, and fulfilling lives.

Thank you for joining me on this journey and may you and your dog enjoy many happy meals together for years to come.

BONUS 1
Behaviour Modification Plans

Behaviour modification is an essential aspect of dog ownership, as it allows owners to address and manage unwanted behaviours effectively. Whether it's excessive barking, destructive chewing, or separation anxiety, understanding the principles of behaviour modification can help owners shape their dog's behaviour in a positive and lasting way. In this chapter, we will explore the key components of behaviour modification plans and provide practical strategies for addressing common behavioural issues.

Understanding Behaviour Modification:

Behaviour modification is a systematic approach to changing a dog's behaviour through positive reinforcement, redirection, and consistency. It involves identifying the underlying causes of undesirable behaviours and implementing targeted strategies to encourage desired behaviours instead. The goal is not just to suppress unwanted behaviours temporarily but to promote long-term behaviour change and improve the overall well-being of the dog.

Key Components of Behaviour Modification Plans:

1. **Identifying the Behaviour:** The first step in creating a behaviour modification plan is to identify the specific behaviour that needs to be addressed. This may involve observing the dog's behaviour closely, keeping a behaviour journal, and consulting with a professional dog trainer or behaviorist if needed.

2. **Understanding Triggers:** Once the behaviour is identified, it's essential to understand what triggers or reinforces it. Triggers can be environmental factors, such as loud noises or unfamiliar people, or internal factors, such as fear or anxiety. By identifying triggers, owners can implement strategies to manage or avoid them.

3. **Setting Clear Goals:** Establishing clear and achievable goals is crucial for success in behaviour modification. Owners should define what specific behaviours they want to change or eliminate and what replacement behaviours they want to encourage. Goals should be realistic, measurable, and tailored to the individual dog's needs and abilities.

4. **Implementing Positive Reinforcement:** Positive reinforcement involves rewarding desired behaviours with praise, treats, toys, or other rewards. By rewarding good behaviour, owners can encourage their dogs to repeat it in the future. It's essential to be consistent with reinforcement and to reward the behaviour immediately after it occurs.

5. **Redirecting Unwanted Behaviours:** Rather than punishing or scolding unwanted behaviours, owners should focus on redirecting them towards more appropriate alternatives. This may involve teaching the dog incompatible behaviours or providing alternative outlets for their energy and instincts.

6. **Consistency and Patience:** Consistency is key to successful behaviour modification. Owners must be consistent in their training methods, expectations, and responses to their dog's behaviour. It's also essential to be patient and understanding, as behaviour change takes time and effort.

Common Behaviour Modification Strategies:

1. **Desensitization and Counterconditioning:** This involves gradually exposing the dog to the trigger at a low intensity while pairing it with something positive, such as treats or play. Over time, the dog learns to associate the trigger with positive experiences and becomes less reactive.

2. **Training Alternative Behaviours:** Teaching the dog alternative behaviours that are incompatible with the unwanted behaviour can be an effective way to redirect their focus. For example, teaching a dog to sit or lie down instead of jumping up on visitors.

3. **Management and Environmental Changes:** Making changes to the dog's environment can help prevent unwanted behaviours from occurring. This may involve using baby gates to restrict access to certain areas, providing plenty of mental and physical stimulation, and removing or securing items that the dog may be tempted to chew or destroy.

4. **Gradual Exposure:** For dogs with fears or phobias, gradual exposure to the fearful stimulus in a controlled and positive way can help them overcome their fears. This may involve starting with very low-intensity exposure and gradually increasing the intensity over time as the dog becomes more comfortable.

5. **Seeking Professional Help:** In some cases, behaviour modification may require the assistance of a professional dog trainer or behaviorist. These professionals can provide personalized guidance and support based on the dog's individual needs and circumstances.

Behaviour modification is a powerful tool for shaping a dog's behaviour and promoting a harmonious relationship between dogs and their owners. By understanding the principles of behaviour modification and implementing targeted strategies, owners can effectively address unwanted behaviours and foster positive behaviour change in their dogs. With patience, consistency, and positive reinforcement, nearly any behaviour can be modified, leading to a happier and more well-behaved canine companion.

REVIEW PAGE

Thank you for choosing to embark on this journey with me through the pages of **"LOW-CARB DOG FOOD AND TREATS COOKBOOK"** Your decision to invest in my work means the world to me, and I am deeply grateful for your support.

As an author, there's nothing quite as rewarding as knowing that my words have resonated with someone like you. Now that you've experienced the story, I would greatly appreciate your feedback. Your honest review is not only invaluable in helping me grow as a writer but also serves as a source of motivation to continue creating.

Please consider leaving a honest review on my book by scanning the barcode below it will take you to my Author central page you can find the book and leave a review.

Your support and encouragement mean everything to me. Thank you for being a part of this journey.

BONUS 2
30 Day Meal Plan

Day	Breakfast	Lunch	Dinner	Treats
1	Scrambled eggs with spinach	Grilled chicken breast with green beans	Turkey and vegetable stew	Carrot sticks
2	Salmon and asparagus omelette	Turkey and pumpkin stew	Beef and broccoli stir-fry	Frozen blueberries
3	Chicken and zucchini frittata	Beef and spinach meatballs	Chicken and sweet potato casserole	Apple slices
4	Turkey and cauliflower rice bowl	Salmon and green bean bake	Beef and cabbage stew	Green beans
5	Egg muffins with diced turkey	Chicken and broccoli chowder	Turkey and lentil stew	Banana slices
6	Spinach and cheese omelette	Beef and butternut squash soup	Salmon and cauliflower soup	Cottage cheese
7	Turkey and carrot muffins	Chicken and spinach salad	Beef and sweet potato stew	Watermelon cubes

8	Scrambled eggs with bell peppers	Turkey and vegetable stir-fry	Beef and cabbage stir-fry	Peanut butter on celery sticks
9	Salmon and zucchini scramble	Beef and broccoli casserole	Chicken and pumpkin soup	Frozen green peas
10	Chicken and kale frittata	Turkey and green bean stew	Salmon and sweet potato chowder	Broccoli florets
11	Egg muffins with diced chicken	Beef and spinach stir-fry	Turkey and cauliflower stew	Plain yogurt with strawberries
12	Spinach and cheese omelette	Chicken and asparagus bake	Beef and carrot stew	Celery sticks with almond butter
13	Turkey and mushroom scramble	Salmon and broccoli casserole	Chicken and zucchini stew	Cantaloupe chunks
14	Scrambled eggs with diced turkey	Beef and cauliflower rice bowl	Turkey and green bean casserole	Frozen raspberries
15	Salmon and spinach omelette	Chicken and cauliflower soup	Beef and asparagus stir-fry	Cucumber slices
16	Chicken and bell pepper scramble	Turkey and kale salad	Salmon and butternut squash stew	Carrot and apple slices

17	Egg muffins with diced beef	Beef and green bean stir-fry	Chicken and sweet potato bake	Plain yogurt with blueberries
18	Spinach and cheese frittata	Chicken and cabbage soup	Turkey and broccoli casserole	Green peas
19	Turkey and zucchini scramble	Salmon and cauliflower bake	Beef and spinach stew	Watermelon slices
20	Scrambled eggs with diced chicken	Beef and broccoli casserole	Chicken and carrot stew	Celery sticks with peanut butter
21	Salmon and asparagus omelette	Turkey and sweet potato bake	Beef and green bean stir-fry	Frozen strawberries
22	Chicken and spinach frittata	Beef and cauliflower stew	Salmon and zucchini casserole	Apple slices with almond butter
23	Egg muffins with diced turkey	Chicken and broccoli stir-fry	Turkey and asparagus bake	Carrot sticks with cottage cheese
24	Spinach and cheese omelette	Salmon and green bean stew	Beef and mushroom stir-fry	Frozen peas
25	Turkey and cauliflower scramble	Beef and spinach meatballs	Chicken and bell pepper bake	Blueberries

26	Scrambled eggs with diced beef	Chicken and zucchini stew	Turkey and kale soup	Cucumber slices with cream cheese
27	Salmon and broccoli omelette	Beef and carrot casserole	Chicken and cauliflower stir-fry	Cantaloupe chunks with cottage cheese
28	Chicken and bell pepper scramble	Turkey and asparagus stir-fry	Beef and broccoli bake	Watermelon cubes with peanut butter
29	Egg muffins with diced chicken	Salmon and cauliflower rice bowl	Turkey and mushroom stew	Frozen raspberries with plain yogurt
30	Spinach and cheese frittata	Chicken and sweet potato stew	Beef and green bean casserole	Carrot sticks with hummus

MEAL PLANNER JOURNAL

Meal Planner

Week of:

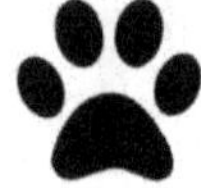

Monday		
BREAKFAST		
LUNCH		
DINNER		
SNACK		

Tuesday		
BREAKFAST		
LUNCH		
DINNER		
SNACK		

Wednesday		
BREAKFAST		
LUNCH		
DINNER		
SNACK		

Thursday		
BREAKFAST		
LUNCH		
DINNER		
SNACK		

Friday		
BREAKFAST		
LUNCH		
DINNER		
SNACK		

Saturday		
BREAKFAST		
LUNCH		
DINNER		
SNACK		

Sunday		
BREAKFAST		
LUNCH		
DINNER		
SNACK		

NOTES:

Meal Planner

Week of:

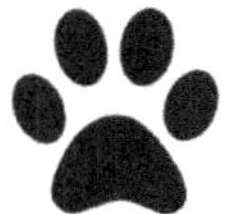

Monday

BREAKFAST

LUNCH

DINNER

SNACK

Tuesday

BREAKFAST

LUNCH

DINNER

SNACK

Wednesday

BREAKFAST

LUNCH

DINNER

SNACK

Thursday

BREAKFAST

LUNCH

DINNER

SNACK

Friday

BREAKFAST

LUNCH

DINNER

SNACK

Saturday

BREAKFAST

LUNCH

DINNER

SNACK

Sunday

BREAKFAST

LUNCH

DINNER

SNACK

NOTES:

Meal Planner

Week of:

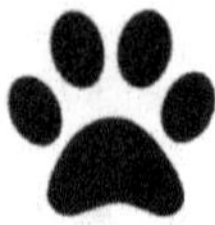

Monday

BREAKFAST

LUNCH

DINNER

SNACK

Tuesday

BREAKFAST

LUNCH

DINNER

SNACK

Wednesday

BREAKFAST

LUNCH

DINNER

SNACK

Thursday

BREAKFAST

LUNCH

DINNER

SNACK

Friday

BREAKFAST

LUNCH

DINNER

SNACK

Saturday

BREAKFAST

LUNCH

DINNER

SNACK

Sunday

BREAKFAST

LUNCH

DINNER

SNACK

NOTES:

Meal Planner

Week of:

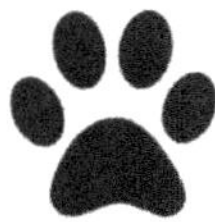

Monday

BREAKFAST

LUNCH

DINNER

SNACK

Tuesday

BREAKFAST

LUNCH

DINNER

SNACK

Wednesday

BREAKFAST

LUNCH

DINNER

SNACK

Thursday

BREAKFAST

LUNCH

DINNER

SNACK

Friday

BREAKFAST

LUNCH

DINNER

SNACK

Saturday

BREAKFAST

LUNCH

DINNER

SNACK

Sunday

BREAKFAST

LUNCH

DINNER

SNACK

NOTES:

Meal Planner

Week of:

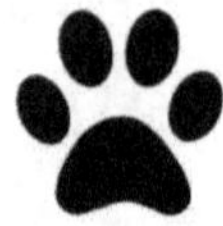

Monday	**Tuesday**	**Wednesday**
BREAKFAST	BREAKFAST	BREAKFAST
LUNCH	LUNCH	LUNCH
DINNER	DINNER	DINNER
SNACK	SNACK	SNACK
Thursday	**Friday**	**Saturday**
BREAKFAST	BREAKFAST	BREAKFAST
LUNCH	LUNCH	LUNCH
DINNER	DINNER	DINNER
SNACK	SNACK	SNACK

Sunday	NOTES:
BREAKFAST	
LUNCH	
DINNER	
SNACK	

Meal Planner

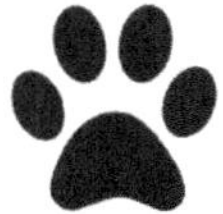

Week of:

Monday	**Tuesday**	**Wednesday**
BREAKFAST	BREAKFAST	BREAKFAST
LUNCH	LUNCH	LUNCH
DINNER	DINNER	DINNER
SNACK	SNACK	SNACK
Thursday	**Friday**	**Saturday**
BREAKFAST	BREAKFAST	BREAKFAST
LUNCH	LUNCH	LUNCH
DINNER	DINNER	DINNER
SNACK	SNACK	SNACK

Sunday	NOTES:
BREAKFAST	
LUNCH	
DINNER	
SNACK	

Meal Planner

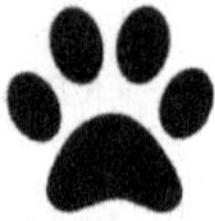

Week of:

Monday	**Tuesday**	**Wednesday**
BREAKFAST	BREAKFAST	BREAKFAST
LUNCH	LUNCH	LUNCH
DINNER	DINNER	DINNER
SNACK	SNACK	SNACK
Thursday	**Friday**	**Saturday**
BREAKFAST	BREAKFAST	BREAKFAST
LUNCH	LUNCH	LUNCH
DINNER	DINNER	DINNER
SNACK	SNACK	SNACK

Sunday	NOTES:
BREAKFAST	
LUNCH	
DINNER	
SNACK	

Meal Planner

Week of:

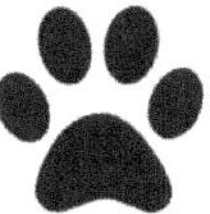

Monday	**Tuesday**	**Wednesday**
BREAKFAST	BREAKFAST	BREAKFAST
LUNCH	LUNCH	LUNCH
DINNER	DINNER	DINNER
SNACK	SNACK	SNACK
Thursday	**Friday**	**Saturday**
BREAKFAST	BREAKFAST	BREAKFAST
LUNCH	LUNCH	LUNCH
DINNER	DINNER	DINNER
SNACK	SNACK	SNACK

Sunday	NOTES:
BREAKFAST	
LUNCH	
DINNER	
SNACK	

Meal Planner

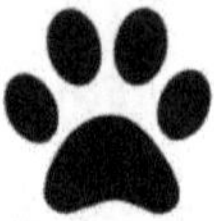

Week of:

Monday	**Tuesday**	**Wednesday**
BREAKFAST	BREAKFAST	BREAKFAST
LUNCH	LUNCH	LUNCH
DINNER	DINNER	DINNER
SNACK	SNACK	SNACK
Thursday	**Friday**	**Saturday**
BREAKFAST	BREAKFAST	BREAKFAST
LUNCH	LUNCH	LUNCH
DINNER	DINNER	DINNER
SNACK	SNACK	SNACK

Sunday	NOTES:
BREAKFAST	
LUNCH	
DINNER	
SNACK	

Meal Planner

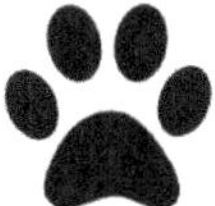

Week of:

Monday

BREAKFAST

LUNCH

DINNER

SNACK

Tuesday

BREAKFAST

LUNCH

DINNER

SNACK

Wednesday

BREAKFAST

LUNCH

DINNER

SNACK

Thursday

BREAKFAST

LUNCH

DINNER

SNACK

Friday

BREAKFAST

LUNCH

DINNER

SNACK

Saturday

BREAKFAST

LUNCH

DINNER

SNACK

Sunday

BREAKFAST

LUNCH

DINNER

SNACK

NOTES:

Meal Planner

Month of:

Sun	Mon	Tues	Wed	Thurs	Fri	Sai